T0193968

ARE YOU EATING ORGANIC

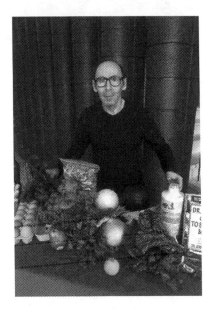

Paul Ciaravella

BALBOA.
PRESS

A DIVISION OF HAY HOUSE

Copyright © 2016 Paul Ciaravella.

All rights reserved. No part of this book may be used or reproduced by any means, graphic, electronic, or mechanical, including photocopying, recording, taping or by any information storage retrieval system without the written permission of the author except in the case of brief quotations embodied in critical articles and reviews.

The information, ideas, and suggestions in this book are not intended as a substitute for professional medical advice. Before following any suggestions contained in this book, you should consult your personal physician. Neither the author nor the publisher shall be liable or responsible for any loss or damage allegedly arising as a consequence of your use or application of any information or suggestions in this book.

Balboa Press books may be ordered through booksellers or by contacting:

Balboa Press
A Division of Hay House
1663 Liberty Drive
Bloomington, IN 47403
www.balboapress.com
1 (877) 407-4847

Because of the dynamic nature of the Internet, any web addresses or links contained in this book may have changed since publication and may no longer be valid. The views expressed in this work are solely those of the author and do not necessarily reflect the views of the publisher, and the publisher hereby disclaims any responsibility for them.

The author of this book does not dispense medical advice or prescribe the use of any technique as a form of treatment for physical, emotional, or medical problems without the advice of a physician, either directly or indirectly. The intent of the author is only to offer information of a general nature to help you in your quest for emotional and spiritual well-being. In the event you use any of the information in this book for yourself, which is your constitutional right, the author and the publisher assume no responsibility for your actions.

Any people depicted in stock imagery provided by Getty Images are models, and such images are being used for illustrative purposes only. Certain stock imagery © Getty Images.

Print information available on the last page.

ISBN: 978-1-9822-2221-5 (sc)
ISBN: 978-1-9822-2222-2 (e)

Balboa Press rev. date: 05/13/2019

Table of Contents

FOREWORD

Organic foods are in demand due to toxicity in our soils.

Many illnesses are on the rise, including allergies, diabetes, autism, Parkinson's and mental illness, just to name a few. Many of these can be blamed on environmental issues. We have lost 40% of the oxygen in the atmosphere due to polluting our oceans. They have become very acidic, losing 5% of their alkalinity, such that our drinking water must be filtered. Our soils are depleted. The last hundred years, we have been growing crops and never mineralizing back.

All we have to do is take care of this planet a little better with the little things and God will take care of the rest with the rain and snow, the oxygen, the sky, the winds, the volcanoes, the soils, the oceans, the air. This is a living live planet, we must be on guard and aware.

Our future demands change; we have to clean up our act.

Paul Ciaravella, Author

Chapter 1

A WARNING TO VEGETARIANS

I wrote this chapter to warn you about becoming vegetarian.

Should you find yourself to be tired of everything...the usual routine meats, barbeques, stews processed meats, broiled, baked...you've had enough. Next morning, you decide to become a vegetarian. I don't blame you.

The first thing you have to learn is that vegetables have a lot of pesticides. You also have to learn something about organic foods. Even though there is a ban on these chemicals, farmers still buy them. And, farmers are exempt from them, which means that farmers are still spraying pesticides. Herbicides are one of the reasons crops grow faster. As a result of crops growing faster, farmers may show a profit.

In reality, I met with a few farmers and asked about their farming operations, one farmer told me that the bank loan has to be paid on time. The pressure is on loans, where they have this monthly commitment that has to be honoured. He said organics take longer to grow and we would go bankrupt. Even though there is a ban on pesticides, farmers are exempt. Our government is helping the banks and the farmers, rather than helping us with what we eat. We are not eating by choice. For this reason, we have to educate ourselves about organics before deciding to become a vegetarian. I talk more about organics chapter 3.

While I write this book, I am reminded of the first book that I wrote, *Shaken but in Control*, which is mostly about chemicals, pesticides, herbicides, fungicides, additives, DDT, lead, preservatives, mercury, misleading us into mental illness. All I am really concerned about is eating clean foods not sprayed with anything toxic.

I have the freedom to choose, no one chooses for me.

We live under a system where we have the freedom to choose. Then, why are you choosing for me? However you have the right to choose vegetarian or carnivore, coffee or tea.

This book is written for those people who are skeptical about organic foods. I hope you will find it to be one of the most exciting and knowledgeable guides on organic foods and of the author's personal experience and skills. It is a "must read".

Your health is a gift...you earn your diseases.
Your diploma can be whatever you earned...I
graduated with Parkinson's and I looked after my
body better than anyone. - Paul Ciaravella

Chapter 2

EAT YOUR FOOD, DON'T THROW IT OUT

Some things have value, like food preparation. We don't pay attention with what we use and sometimes foods are discarded or misused by mistake or by lack of knowledge or ignorance.

For example, we peel the potatoes and the peels we throw out. Why, I ask? Potato peels have nutrition. Under the skin, you will find natural sodium, good for all your joints, stomach lining, and eyes. The explanation is simple, where the blood doesn't reach, the sodium will. Manmade sodium chloride - you don't want to use it - the second ingredient is sugar. In a watermelon, the top red part that we eat is very cleansing and soothing. However, did you know that the bottom white part contains chlorine and sodium, both excellent cleansers? Another mineral routinely thrown out is calcium, found in beet tops and the leaves we cut off. Grapes contain seeds; we eat the grapes and throw out the seeds. If you were to chew them, you would find their taste bitter. What you are tasting is potassium, which is good for natural bowel movement. Potassium is one mineral that we need to have plenty of at all times.

Out all this good stuff goes to the recycle bin. The bin is healthy, not us.

We eat Almonds, which are very rich in calcium, iron, manganese, potassium, phosphorus and carbon nitrogen, but unless you soak them overnight in water, you won't digest them properly and then you will have to chew them at least 20 times. Another thing we don't do properly; Raisins should be revived in hot water for a few minutes. This way, the amount of sugar released to you at once is reduced. Dry fruit has very high levels of concentrated sugar. It'll be a sugar shock, but if there was a bee or a wasp laying their eggs, the hot water would kill the eggs originally laid there by insects.

Ask any nutritionist what they most desire; he or she will say more organic foods or biodynamics
- Paul Ciaravella

Chapter 3

PLU CODES

Might as well start this chapter on a strong note It is 4 am and I can't sleep and many things are itching me.

I am still having pesticides in my body and retail stores are pushing foods on us containing chemicals. I don't know why are they doing this to us, but my guess is that they are making a living.

Have you ever wondered why on your fruit there is a little label with a 4 or 5 digit number, some starting with a 4 or a 3, some with a 9 or an 8? Those are called PLU codes. Also, if it is conventional or organic In this fashion, the authorities see that producers are obeying the law and it will be business as usual.

These little labels are numbered, the first number representing whether it is organic or conventional. Before we get there, I must tell you about these codes.

PLU stands for Price Look Up Codes and IFPS stands for International Federation for Produce Standards.

Here is a breakdown of these little stickers on the fruits and vegetables. On organic and biodynamic, it will be a 5 digit number starting with 9, standing for certified organic.

PLU 4 and PLU 3 (the most used) are conventional, I have to be careful, no chemicals whatsoever in my diet or I will suffer more.

However the labelling of GMO foods is not enforced I have yet to see a 5 digit PLU sticker with a leading number of 8 (meaning GMO). Most foods are genetically modified (including soya and corn which are 100% GMO). The truth is out; then what are we hiding? Every store that I go to, the foods are GMO, so why no stickers?[1]

To be safe, remember the code on fruits and vegetables using this simple rhyme:

9 Is fine. Organic. ☺

---

[1] There is no mandatory labeling of genetically engineered foods in Canada despite intensive pubic campaigning and 20 years of polling that consistently show over 80% of Canadians want these labels. Instead, a national standard for voluntary labeling was established - but this is voluntary and no company has yet labeled their products as containing GE ingredients!
64 countries around the world have some type of mandatory labeling GE food law including the European Union, Japan, Australia, Brazil, Russia and China.
An Ipsos Reid poll commissioned by CBAN in September 2015 found that 88% of consumers in Canada want labelling. - Source Canadian Biotechnology Action Network website.

Chapter 4

THE ENVIRONMENT

By now, we know that in the winter months our country, Canada, is cold. During this time, we must import food from other countries.
The City of Toronto is one of the receiving port terminals for all imported foods, coming here by air, trucks, rail and sea.

If the target is the Toronto port, then own food is travelling the following miles.

....New Zealand is 8,760 miles
....Australia is 10,165 miles
....South Africa is 8,200 miles
....Taiwan-China-Japan is 6,430 miles
....India is 7,785 miles
....Israel is 5,800 miles
....Italy-Spain-Greece is 4,970 miles
....The Philippines is 8,300 miles
....Chile is 5,500 miles
....California is 2,175 miles
....México is 2,750 miles
....Saskatchewan in Western Canada is 1,275 miles
....Germany, Austria, France, Portugal, Morocco, Central Europe - the list goes on.

It travels a long way, it doesn't matter if it is organic or not.

I was watching a report on TV where they were saying our Canadian dollar is causing (fresh) fruits and vegetables prices to go up. The word "fresh" was mentioned. Is it really fresh? How in the world can it be fresh?

Environmentally, it isn't worth it, we add too much to overall pollution. These are the bulk of our partner countries that supply us foods and contribute a great deal to pollution of the environment. Our officials allow these activities to happen. You, the reader, do the math. The fuel used is incredible. If you are concerned about lowering pollution levels, write to your Prime Minister and ask him, "What happened to cutting down gas emissions?" Therefore, as a result, we get foods with pesticides, genetically modified....# and pollution.# The problem is that there is a blind eye to the destination which is far away, no one to investigate them and keep loyal and fair trade partner countries in place. This is a wakeup call to politicians, and it is a no brainer to solve. The solution is to keep this model, but have countries rotate every three months and police them. We have to kick countries out of our food supply chain, the ones that take advantage of us instead of shipping us proper foods.

Did you know that some farmers get as little as 6 cents for a pineapple, they pay their staff low labor and live very poorly themselves?

Traveling in the USA domestically or internationally. On average, there are approximately 90,000 daily flights originating from about 9,000 airports around the world, being flown by about 30,000 airplanes. At any given time, there are between 8,000 and 13,000 planes in the air around the globe.

Chapter 5

WHEN PEOPLE CONNECT

Recently, I took an interest in people's habits and some of the things like foods, drinks, snacks, organics, socializing, nutrition, couples, husbands and wives, boyfriends and girlfriends, and families.

A funny thing happened one day. There was a couple sitting at the next table to me at a restaurant in which I was dining. I noticed something... they weren't talking to each other. The husband was looking to the left and the wife was looking to the right. Their body language said it all. I observed wedding bands and felt they were married to each other. Throughout the entire meal, no one spoke a word. One of them ate only organic foods, the other didn't. All of a sudden, there was a conversation about the food. A miracle happened; they were speaking to one another! One of them complained that the food had no nutrition, it wasn't organic, it was full of pesticides. I couldn't help but overhear this conversation. I felt connected with the person that ate only organic food. Yes, they had something in common...food. Sure, food is important, but there are other things to talk about, like the children, travel, house repairs, sports, a bit of gossip. There are many things to discuss at dinner.

Boy, when you are totally discontented and disconnected and have nothing in common, it's marriage melt down time. That is really sad, how does this happen? Too many distractions, maybe TV, maybe simply fallout. There are times when a relationship is failing and you disconnect. It is hard work to find a way to restore and reconnect with your mate.

Sometimes foods play a negative role and you can make it positive with organics. You can't go wrong, your soul and heart will be at peace. Your stress levels will come down, trust me, I have gone through this a few times with loved ones.

What can I say? If you start eating organic, I promise you, in ninety days, your body won't feel as hungry, because conventional foods have less nutrition than organic (more on this later). Since I improved my nutrition, my skin looks better, I'm not as hungry any more, and I have more energy.

Your loved ones can make a lot difference in your love for foods and influence. Be careful, if you must eat with them, are they organic? –
Paul Ciaravella

Chapter 6

BACK ON TOP

Most people today complain that organic foods are too expensive, but yet the lottery sector is grabbing their funds left and right, any which way they can. I hear people say we can't afford shopping today, especially organic foods, but they will go and buy tobacco products, fast foods, lottery tickets, junk food, candy, expensive shoes and clothing, and big ticket autos. Let me remind you, organic foods will help more than you think. Of course; don't forget about what system we live under, with the power to choose.

I ask these people a simple question. "Do you know that our soil has been depleted for many years?" Our soil is missing key components, such as calcium, magnesium, manganese, iron, silicon, nitrogen, potassium, sodium, phosphorus and many others. Another question? "Do you supplement your food?" Most the time the answer is "What do you mean?" I reply, "You know, supplement them with vitamins and minerals." The answer is invariably no. When I ask why not, they say that they eat healthy. I love this, this is my favorite answer. Then I ask "What does eating healthy mean?" They have no clue. This means the individual lacks food skills, how to buy it, where to find it, and the habit of saving for the entire lifestyle. I meet so many people like this. One of the reasons I am sharing this information with you is to help you capture the energy that you once had and bring back a vibrant lifestyle.

You can go without vitamins for a while, but you need to have your daily supplements. Ask any naturopathic doctor, he or she will give you an explanation about supplementing with minerals.

I was depleted for the longest time - mineral deficient. One day I found myself reading a book called *Vibrant Health from Your Kitchen,* by Dr. Bernard Jensen. He explained in his book that if you are low in minerals, it could affect your attitude, feelings of love, sex, and energy levels.

That's the point at which I started to think about eating organic. According to professional food growers, biodynamic soils contain more minerals. I jumped on this new information. Dr. Jensen gave tips on how to find them. He gave an example of a" farmer who had an issue with his herd of goats" In the spring, shortly after the babies were born, the mothers would abandon them. They simply refused to claim them. The story goes on to say that after trying supplements for the goats, a breakthrough happened. They discovered the land was contaminated, their soil was missing a key mineral; it had very low levels of manganese. After they started feeding this mineral to the goats, the mothers were claiming back their young. The farmer was thrilled about this discovery - how a simple unknown mineral such as manganese made a bunch of goats happy.

Manganese produces astonishing results. This mineral now has a nickname - "the love element". Maybe we should supply an abundance of the mineral manganese to people going through a divorce. Maybe there would be hope and a future for them. Maybe by introducing this love element, they would be back on top once again. On the other hand, this could bankrupt divorce lawyers.

Can you imagine what kind of people we would have; nicer folks these days are rare. We live in a toxic world, we should give a try. Why not?

Manganese is found in these foods and to name almonds, apples, apricots, green beans, blackberries, butternut squash, celery, walnuts, oats, and olives. If you know of any more foods containing this mineral, particularly in other parts of the world, please send me an email and I will add them to the list.

These foods must be organic; their main function is for the brain and nerves to function. I stumbled across this information by accident. In 2008, when I was diagnosed with Parkinson's, I was desperate to learn everything I could. I started to have tremors on the back of my head and legs. Now, everything seems to be okay. Thanks to all my supporters that stood by me, you know who you are.

I named this chapter Back on Top. When you find yourself in crisis, the first symptom is depression. I have been there, don't let them tell you that you have depression. So what should you do? Get up in the morning and jump up and down and say "I am so excited I have Parkinson's (or diabetes) (or cancer)? No. it's an obvious thing. Of course, you are depressed. But, be careful, don't let it control your life. You can only drown if you stay in the water. Come out, dry yourself off and get back on top of your life again.

I always thought that rich people never had problems, only the poor. Boy, was I wrong! Coming from an average family, most of us didn't know any rich people. Somewhere, some day, we hope to strike it rich, although most of us have learned to be content with what we have now.

The author often mentions that we have to grow and try to be ready to become a real man. If are not yet ready to be men, then what are we? We are people with hopes and dreams, hoping the future will bring us success and happiness. I started looking at life differently, outside of the box. I made a decision; this was the day to march on and to lay down a plan of action; I wanted to have a goal, a direction. Remember, most of us are poor navigators but we are in control.

Look ahead and see as much you can see and keep looking until you cannot see any more. This exercise worked for me. Let's say you want to lose twenty pounds - you have to visualize that you are going to look good.

See what I mean? Difficult isn't it? Well, our goals are the same. Visualize all of your dreams and the confidence level will rise like the sun. You'll be back.

Once you have done that, things will improve tremendously for the future. What do you have to lose?

Often people ask me, "How are you, Paul?" My reply is humorous. I say "If I was any better, my health wouldn't be able to stand it." I say it with pride. Now you know how I feel. I decided that Back on Top is my favorite chapter. The reason why is, I have been battling Parkinson's since 2008. Parkinson's is not a disease, but an environmental neurotransmitter challenge. I went down into depression originally for obvious reasons. Then with family pressures, I started to use the medicines that the traditional doctors prescribed, but there was no improvement until I met a retired MD, Dr. Deborah Drake. She was very helpful, very smart and knew nutrition like nobody's business. After doing my own research, everything she told me made sense. In fact, many people wanted to know what I was taking in terms of supplements and asked "Where is your book?" This is what inspired me to write my very first book, *Shaken but in Control.*

To get to the top, there are rules; things like a strong body, healthy brain and some kind of knowledge about organic foods.

A garden without planning would look really messed up. The other area is learning about becoming a certified organic member. You must be able to fertilize to produce good crops and foods with value.

It wasn't until that I started to see and understand how heavy metals are stored in the body that the pieces started to fit together. The question was, where in the body are they stored? The brain? Maybe the feet? The liver, the other organs? I was looking for an answer within myself. With research and help from other people, these are the things that I found out. The brain, the liver and the feet provide good storage for heavy metals, the feet more so, because of gravity. Makes sense. Where do they come from? Air pollution, mercury, lead from water pipes, environments, molds, dusts and so on.

When you go to sleep at night and you are lying down flat, your blood circulates throughout the body, rotating all night and our liver is working around the clock to cleanse our blood. Doctors say that this organ cleanses up to 540 gallons of blood each and every day. The solution on cleansing the feet and minimizing heavy metals is in a later chapter. I don't endorse any products yet. But I will give you some tips on how to detox the feet using salts to do the job. Symptoms of heavy metals in the feet are: sore, wet, smelly feet; cracked skin; headaches and very painful skin.

Sometimes it might be parasites in the feet causing extra toxins. We use the toilet to eliminate, they use our body and most of the time we have extra toxins to eliminate - more work for the liver. I was able to detox my liver and my feet and felt fantastic afterwards; using alka-bath salts with gem stones for my feet and Liver Master for my liver.

Dealing with Parkinson's, I am always on the lookout for foods, spices, herbs, minerals, vitamins; remedies that work for me. One of the reasons I am certified organic is that I want to pay attention. The present and future is where it's at; we have to learn to respect our bodies. Tell your friends and family to have some understanding that your food should be pure, whole and fresh, and most importantly, certified organic.

All these positive and negative situations are part of life; they arise daily and we have to deal with the real key is that it is never what happens, rather what you do about it, and how you handle things. The way you see yourself is how other people see you. To be on top of situations, you need to get physically fit, mentally sharp, spiritually alive and loaded with a plan of action. This is an attitude, most valuable and important to all of us; our performance depends on it. Cheer up.

People don't have it in them to be on top; you must learn or develop these skills.

"But Paul", you say, "How I can do it?" In my opinion, read books. You say, "Paul, I don't have time, if you worked where I work, fight the traffic etc. etc. etc."

Too bad it is a true fact that most people have these excuses and can't be back on top, rather remain at the bottom with their health and also financial freedom. It is not a good way to live, with no knowledge and poor habits.

My response is, you have enough time to eat supper, drink something, watch a little TV and go to bed, the next day it is same old thing all over again. You speak the language of the poor. You've got to get excited to be back on top, learn about dreaming things like staying healthy, no illness. Learn about organic foods, pesticides, preservatives, nasty chemicals in cosmetics, clean foods, minerals, vitamins, supplements, oils, fats, the trace minerals, the macro minerals, enzymes, probiotics, antioxidants, algae, herbs, detoxifications, being vibrant and how to get there. Learn about being alkaline versus acidic, about water, about which foods are good for you.

I encourage you to read *Vibrant Health from Your Kitchen* and some other books on health (listed at the end of the book). Think and grow rich, instead of not thinking and growing poor. You will feel better, more confident about yourself and you will save money.

Render more service than that for which you are paid, and you will soon be paid for more than you render. The law of "Increasing Returns" takes care of this! -
The Law of Success - Napoleon Hill

Chapter 7

ARE YOU EATING ORGANIC NOW?

Are you eating organic now? If not, then you are eating. Back in the 70's, organic foods were introduced in Toronto. As a matter of fact, there were very few health food stores and hardly any information on natural products. When coming out of a health food store, if people saw you, they called you a" health freak", a "limy". Those days were tough; People did not welcome natural health. In the 80's and 90's, things became easier as people started to tolerate this trend more and more. Now, many people are asking the famous line, "Is it organic?"

I just finished participating in a health show called Whole Life Expo, one of the largest health shows in the country. Canada now has several shows of this nature. What a difference from 1970 to today, you can enter a health food store freely and come out with ease and no criticism!

Ontario is leading with over 2,000 stores and many farmers going towards organics. It is nice to see that; maybe there is a God after all.

Most people that I talk with want to know if organic food is better than conventional. My answer to this question is two part; if it is not sprayed with chemicals and if it is grown in soil.

If is grown in hydroponics, with water and chemicals, yes it is organic, but it doesn't have the rich minerals to supply your body what it needs. Therefore, you are buying a very expensive food with no nutrition. So ask questions, if it is important to you. Where and how was it grown?

Conventional foods are 40% lower in nutrition. One of the reasons is that the land is neglected by the farmers. Do they think that God is going to rain minerals?

Water sold in stores is the biggest hype and some very good marketing tactics are used to sell water. Did you ever wonder why they call it mineral water? I sent a bottle to a lab. The results showed came back; there were no minerals!

Do I have to be a watch dog?

Where am I going with this? Simple, ask questions.

....I often wonder about Coca Cola they call one of their products Diet Coke. Is it coke or a die.t, which one is it?
....Drywall - does this mean the wall is dry or the wall is wet? The name is confusing, another way to sell product.

There are other products....

....Spring roll - is it a spring or is it a roll?
....Cream of wheat - is it cream or is it a wheat
....Lipstick - is it lip or is a stick? By the way did you know that a woman uses up to 5 pounds of lipstick in her life?
....Hot dog - what is it, a dog that is very hot?
....Eggplant - is an egg or a plant?
....Gift card - is it a gift or is it a card?
....Minute rice - is it a minute or rice?
....Parkway - is it a park or a way?

By now, you can tell I am not slandering products of marketing merely having some fun with the way products are worded.

....Chicken balls - I didn't know that chickens had balls.

....The drinks are on the house - should I go outside to see if the drinks are on the house?

....Some others would say the drinks are on me.

....Stores issues rainchecks - is it rain or a check?

....Website - is it a web or is it a site?

....Extra virgin olive oil - what is it, a virgin or an oil?

....Mineral water - is it water or a mineral?

....Vitamin water - what is it a vitamin or a water?

You catch my drift.

Learning about nutrition requires some understanding of the English language and also some of these marketing tactics. That way, we don't get cheated. Larger stores need to teach their purchasing agents how to buy organic foods; otherwise, some dishonest seller can and will cheat them. We will be defrauded, as well, because their buying skills were poor. Makes sense.

I once bought organic apples; on my first bite, my lips were burning. The store has a good reputation, somehow they got cheated.

Also, stores that carry both conventional and organic products should be certified by me or some nutritional school that teaches them how to buy certified organic. Holistic schools strive to better serve the customers.

Try to eat organically. Some foods are seasonal. What do we do? Where do we shop? My advice is to buy whatever is in season. Don't worry, you won't fall apart.

Learn something about how food is grown.

Take English cucumbers. I don't recommend them because they are grown in hot houses; in the morning, their size is like your baby finger. At 4 pm, they are a foot long. These have some form of pesticides, along with fungicides and fertilizers and are kept in stores with a chemical solution, otherwise they would look old and no one would buy them. Chemicals have been used, but in pickles, cucumbers are safe.

Combining Foods

Legumes are under the radar. Beans can be good or tough on you. They must be organic or your digestive system will be bombarded with unwanted chemicals that are difficult to digest.

Should you be eating them? Now, consider combining all beans and lentils with rice, not with wheat products. For instance, Italians have a recipe "pasta e Faggioli" which means pasta and beans. The Faggioli part is a legume, not a very good mix, but tasty and a traditional food. Try taking rice and Faggioli and test them to see which one is easier to digest. Because it is organic, doesn't mean it is good for you.

There are many foods for us to eat, many are made for vegetarians and some people that prefer a steak. Women tend to prefer other foods, like veggies and fish (don't get me wrong, women like a good steak, too!) Food combining must be mastered for your food to have a positive effect on your body. For example, apple pie and steak, this is a bad combo, sugar and protein. Spaghetti and meatballs or bread with any meats, also a bad combo By the way, we have bread three times a day; toast for breakfast, a sandwich for lunch, for dinner, we might have pizza. Wheat is always present and we eat too much in a meal with protein. My point is, that if every meal is executed in this fashion, our digestive system will back up. It will have so many meals not processed properly, and this will slow down the bowel transit time. Avoid proteins and sugars together or minimize some of them.

I found out that a potato has starch, protein and sugars. The center of the potato is 100% starch, 19 % protein, and 80% sugar. Nature supplied us with this balance, then it must be okay. But, you are manager of your own menu, so make sure you understand it. Meat and potatoes are foods that I like, however I can't process them. My digestion gets all excited with gas and bloating and if I add coffee and desserts, boy, do I know it!

Sometimes you have to listen to your body. Should you get a headache or heartburn, these are signs of indigestion, not because you are lacking Turns®! By the way, Turns® are nothing more than confectionary sugar. For heartburn, try a teaspoon of raw or wild honey...works just as well...OR correct the food originally and avoid the problem.

Meat and potatoes as a combo is not a very good mix, and difficult to digest because it neutralizes, doesn't move down and the digestive system becomes bloated. It was organic all right, but it got stuck up there. To improve it and move forward, eat a piece of pineapple, yellow if possible, and that meal will be saved. Or a piece of watermelon including the white bottom part, which has chlorine and sodium. These are good cleansers, considered "down" foods, which I will explain later on in this chapter. Meat and potatoes are considered "up" foods; what this means is that some foods remain up, some foods go down easy.

The other reason we get bloated is because we drink liquids with our meals. You should drink only if you are choking or 45 minutes after you are done eating to avoid bloating. One of the major influences comes from the large junk food retailers. For example, you go to order a meal from a fast food restaurant takeout menu; combo 1 has food and a large cold drink, ditto for combos 2, 3 and 4.

Cold and hot foods - what are they and how they work, organic or not.

Consider the following chart:

Left - Hot foods	Right - Cold foods
Garlic, onions	Kale, lettuce
Cayenne, ginger	Watermelon
Asparagus, raw milk	Kelp, dulse
Oats, tomatoes	Cucumber, endive
Leeks, chives	Celery, parsley

Garlic, onions, cayenne, red wine, kale and lettuce; these contain sulfur and are considered the heating elements. These foods are good to balance your body in the summer time. Pick a few of each. If you don't, you might be too hot. If you consider only the foods on your left, likewise in the winter, you will shiver.

If you choose all foods on the right, they are very simple to tolerate.

These are some of the foods that you can choose to balance hot and cold. If your body always feels cold or hot, eat 50% hot and 50% cold. Trust me, it works. There are many more foods to choose from (please refer to *Vibrant Health from Your Kitchen* by Dr. Bernard Jensen).

I also mentioned earlier that yellow foods will assist with bowel movements. Here is a list of these foods. Yellow beets, watermelon, beans, peaches, apricots, prickly pears, squashes, pumpkins, peppers, millet, cornmeal, polenta, mangoes. These foods will guide you to toward a better elimination. Bananas avocados.

Chapter 8

IS YOUR SOIL ORGANIC?

I believe that all of us should have a garden and grow everything possible. There are many vegetables that can be grown in your backyard.

My ancestors are Sicilian. My grandma called her garden "the **Yardino**". It was a piece of land in a very awkward location, sitting on a downward slope. When we walked down, it was awkward, but the plants were vibrant. The fruits and the vegetables tasted incredible; they still do after all these years.

My grandfather lived to be 97 years old. He had a piece of land south of the town approximately one hour away. He called orto, which means garden, but the geographic name was called Mittraha. The land sat on steep hill and he grew a garden spring and summer. At the time, I was 8 or 9 years old. Looking back now, I think, how in the world did that garden grow with temperatures of 40 to 45 degrees? In this type of climate, nothing in our garden would survive here in Maple, Ontario; I have to water daily or my back yard will go dry and die.

There in Sicily, it doesn't rain in the summer months, it is very hot. How did those vegetables grow? It's a miracle, a phenomenon of Mother Nature.

Perhaps the reason why the food grew so well there was because of the minerals from Mount Etna. The whole island, it doesn't matter where you are, is incredibly rich in minerals. You don't need fertilizers, you've got the volcano.

The other thing I want share is on that the steep hill where my grandfather's garden was located, the soil was multicolored, with white traces of salts you could actually pick out with your hands; the soil was gray brown, hardly any black soil like we have here in Canada. The other thing is that region the weather is so hot, the soil cooks and remains loose and dry. There are no freezing marks. It is also rich in minerals and the fruits and vegetables ripen to full maturity.

Sunshine must be present to obtain Vitamin C. If we pick the fruit too early or green, they will be lacking in Vitamin C. Say Vitamin C is on the fruit. Did you know if oranges are picked green, there is no Vitamin C? But yet, the marketing boards tell us there is Vitamin C in oranges. How can that be? Vitamin D is also obtained from the sun. Don't be afraid to pull up your shirt, show your skin to nature and feed off it.

Chapter 9

ENERGIZE YOUR SOIL WITH PARAMAGNETIC ROCK

This is one of the most important projects of the food chain related to minerals in our foods.

I had an idea one day to import some lava rocks from where volcanoes are. It might seem to be an expensive project, but it's a good one I want to ensure no pesticides are used at all in the soil.

We have 50 active volcanoes. Where are they?

.... Mount Etna in Sicily
.... Mauna Loa and Mauna Kea in Hawaii
.... Mount Vesuvius in Italy
.... Mount Pinatubo in the Philippines,
.... Mount St. Helen and Mount Rainer in the USA
.... Mount peels in the Caribbean
.... ABU in china
.... Acamarchi in Chile
.... Zitacuaro valle De bravo in central Mexico
.... West Crater in Washington USA

Just to name a few

These are but a handful of the over 1,800 volcanoes on our live living planet. Yes, they are far away from us, but the possibilities are enormous.

How do fertilizers and pesticides work? But allergies are escalating to the limit, escalating and why mental health issues, traffic and pollution are absolutely out of control, y the reason why is because we have too many empty calories and mineral deficiencies. Lava is made up of crystals and volcanic glass which bubble as magma gets closer to the surface. Cooling off, it crystallizes into liquid volcanic glass. Chemically, lava is made of these elements - oxygen, silicone, aluminum, iron, calcium, sodium, potassium, magnesium, to name just a few. These lavas from volcanoes are rich in minerals (fertilizers are not). Once ground into a sand form, this can be shipped to farmers to test them out.

We have explore all the possibilities, including mineralized soil, which will produce better results.

Who am I to say if this great idea will work, you ask?

I have a garden in my back yard (I call it **Yardino).** The mineralized rock has been there since 2000. You ought to see it! The vegetables are so vibrant and tasty, they smell so good, everything grows, even the weeds are enjoying themselves, and the kale has reached 6 feet plus this is a breakthrough in gardening, I believe. These lavas spread into our soil will last 100 years or more.

Think about it. Why do you think the creator of this planet put here on earth 1,800 plus volcanoes? To keep us healthy. We must respect that. I just hope this planet holds together with all the activity.

The oceans help us moisten our body and trees the plants. The winds move the clouds. The rain washes the planet and all the other things like forest fires. The sun keeps us warm and grows our fruits and vegetables. Without the sun, oranges and mangos, bananas, apples, apricots, you name it, won't have any vitamin C and D, The sun supplies them both.

Don't complain about the snow, the skiers are not complaining. The weather man is putting you up to all this. Telling you that it is all bad is a form of control, instead of saying today is going to be 60% chance of rain, rather than saying 40% chance of sun. Classic case, glass is half full or half empty.

Our seeds are being controlled. Our soil was put on earth for us to use. No seeds, no harvest. No fruit trees either. All the seeds are being controlled by ultimate greed. Our governments are not paying attention to this. A few corporations have found a way to control all seeds. As a result, we are left without seeds; we have to rent them and return them after use.

For example, you get a 50 pound bag of buckwheat from Koto. You must return the 50 pound bag back to them; it says right on the label, the seed is not for sale (see below). Boy, times have changed!

In this decade, freedom is vanishing from us. What in the world is going on if our seeds can no longer be bought?

The seeds are only available on a rental basis. Our freedom is being jeopardized to such an extent that we have no control. And governments are allowing this? I can't believe that lobbyists and corporation would do this to the people of the land.

Greed is a byproduct of hell, I say.

> **If you don't plan your garden, you weed in the fall. Where were you last spring? Weeds grow automatically with or without your approval**
> -Paul Ciaravella

If you don't eat organic foods then what are you eating pesticides

Speaking of apples, I decided to focus nutritionally on **Vitamin** A. Apples are almost a perfect fruit. Their history goes back to the Egyptian era, even in our religion, for thousands of years, including Adam and Eve. Years ago, apples were used to relieve gout.

There are many varieties of apples. We can have fresh apples all year, also, we can make apple cider, apple sauce, juices, spreads, pies. Some doctors used apples to treat "lazy bowel". When you cook apples, keep the heat low so that the delicate pectin and vitamins will be preserved. Apples are alkaline foods that promote digestion, but we have to be mindful of chemical sprays such as pesticides.

At this point I'd like to talk about **Vitamin A.** Apples have a substantial amount compared to other fruits and vegetables.

Have you noticed when you cut an apple in half the oxygen turns the apple brown. Then you cut another apple in half and it doesn't turn brown. What's going on why I was wandering my self the same thing I found that one is organic and the other isn't some clever scientist found a way to use a chemical. For this to happen one more pesticides to deal with.

"AN APPLE PER A DAY KEEPS THE DOCTOR AWAY" BUT IT DOESN'T KEEP THE NURSE AWAY

Compare the following:

Fruit or Vegetable (1 pound)	Amount of Vitamin A (i.u.)
Apples	360.000
Apricots	11.930
Asparagus	3.430
Avocado	900.000

Beets	22.700
Carrots	48.00
Collard	14.200
Dandelion	61.970
Grapefruit	4.770
Kale	21.950
Lettuce	1.700
Mango	14.000
Papaya	5.320
Peach	5.230
Persimmon	10.080
Pumpkin	5.080
Snap bean	2.400
Spinach	26.450
Squash	11.920
Swiss Chard	10.900
Tomatoes	4.080
Turnip Greens	34.470
Watercress	200.450

Why Vitamin A? We don't get enough of this vitamin. The reason Carbohydrates are way up. Our society is a carbohydrate junky. I encourage you to eat some of the foods listed above, especially greens and carrots (the highest in Vitamin A).Bio Chlorella, which is a single- celled edible alga, is also a good source of vitamin A, having nearly 50.000 IU per hundred grams, high in chlorophyll, Vitamin B 12 and a good source of alkaline. Vitamin A is required in big numbers. To be on the safe- side, get 50.000 IU daily from greens and food. I don't encourage you to consume the synthetic type Greens are the best source.

In winter, we lack Vitamin D from lack of sunshine. We depend on Vitamin A. Children are generally Vitamin A deficient, perhaps because many of the foods that they consume are high in sugars and they don't consume enough greens. If you have children, you know what I am talking about.

It is exciting to know that out there, we have a solution to our food. I call it certified organic foods, or should I say free of chemicals. -Paul Ciaravella

We are all dreaming about tasty and organic vibrant food, especially people with extreme allergies. It feels like my expectations are up. So is my future success, based on good health and exercise, and, of course, vibrant soils.

What is magnetic rock? It is rock from nature. Originally, it was a volcanic rock that was produced by our natural living planet via volcano. Thank you, Mother Nature!

By now, you should get a hint of where I am going with this. Once you put this ground up rock in your backyard garden (it is good for a long time), your vegetables will see a difference in growth. I have had mine now for twenty

Years and my garden looks so healthy I have not put anything else in it so far. Twenty years! This is how long this project has being going on. I am happy not to apply chemicals, herbicides, pesticides or fertilizers. I say that with confidence.

Back when I was learning about magnetic rock, I was told to do an experiment with regular soil and the rock; to get two 16 ounce clear glasses, fill one with regular soil and plant two seeds of your choice; in the other glass, use magnetic rock again with two seeds. Water and keep both under a heat lamp. Surprise! They both came up at the same time ten days because both plants were getting moisture and heat. Yes, they will grow. The difference was that the plants from the magnetic rock soil were taller and very vibrant. They both received the same amount of care, water and heat. That got my attention. I was curious; so why the difference in results? The glass with regular soil was low in minerals; the magnetic rock had plenty of mixed minerals, which gave the young plants more energy to develop and grow vibrant and healthy.

This is the way of the future, folks. Think about it. No chemical or fertilizers.

Each and every year, we dump into our environment all kinds of different chemicals. According to a farmer's report, Canadian and US fanners use an estimated 900 million pounds of pesticides and 22 billion pounds of synthetic fertilizers each year You do the math. Then, add to that herbicides, fungicides, growth regulators and fumigants used to protect foods during shipping and storage.

In his 1987 book, *Diet for a New America,* Dr. John Robbins calculates that the combined tonnage of agricultural chemicals dumped in our environment annually is more than the combined weight of the population of the USA.

Have we gone mad? Let your local farmer know about this and stop this madness.

Chapter 10

ORGANIC FARMING

More and more Canadians and Americans are returning to organically grown foods. The taste is adequate, there are more minerals in them and the people of these countries are learning about clean foods.

Fertilizers should be a thing of the past, let's move on with our lives, say goodbye to allergies and acute health challenges. It's never been a better time to make a change. Let's get out of our comfort zone and improve our foods.

Healthy Naturally did a study on vegetables and found some astonishing results. The mineral content in the organically grown foods was significantly higher than in conventional production.

[2]Mineral Content* of Organically Grown vs. Conventional Chemical Input Production							
	Calcium	Magnesium	Potassium	Sodium	Manganese	Iron	Copper
Snap beans							
Conventional	15.5	14.8	29.1	0.0	2.0	10.0	3.0
Organic	40.5	60.0	99.7	8.6	60.0	2.3	69.0
Cabbage							
Conventional	17.5	15.6	53.7	0.8	2.0	20.0	0.4

---

[2] Data from the Firman Bear report, based on research conducted at Rutgers University - Source Natural Foods Associates, Atlanta, TX.

Organic	60.0	43.6	148.3	20.4	13.0	94.0	48.0
Lettuce							
Conventional	16.0	13.1	53.7	0.0	1.0	9.0	3.0
Organic	71.0	43.6	175.5	12.2	169.0	516.0	60.0
Tomatoes							
Conventional	4.5	4.5	58.6	0.0	1.0	1.0	0.0
Organic	23.0	59.2	148.3	6.5	68.1	1938.0	53.0
Spinach							
Conventional	47.5	46.9	84.0	0.8	1.0	19.0	0.5
Organic	96.0	203.9	257.0	69.5	117.0	1584.0	32.0

*Millequivalents per 100g dry weight trace elements ppm.

If you failed many times to lose weight, keep trying, sooner or later you will succeed via persistence - Paul Ciaravella

Foods that get results. Some people struggle with weight problems, some with allergies, and others cannot gain weight. Some are hungry all the time, others are bloated. Being a Nutrition Counselor myself for several years, I have met all kinds of people and they have one thing in common. What is it? They all eat these foods; fast foods, TV dinners, microwave foods, refined, processed, genetically modified, conventional, frozen and overcooked foods. They get no exercise, take no supplements and don't use tools like water filters, juicers, air filters or food processors.

This is a recipe for failure, health wise. Our nations are built and consumed on these foods.

How can we improve upon them?

First, we should look at **organic foods,** meaning free of chemicals, pesticides, herbicides and fungicides.

Second, **biodynamic foods;** these foods are the cream of the crop because the soil fertility is very effective, seeds fertilize to a natural state, and they are the highest in nutrition. You can get more information at www.biodynamicfood.org.

Third, **foods grown in greenhouses,** Plants should be in soil, not containers with chemicals. There are no minerals in buckets, only in soil, otherwise, you will be buying very expensive food with no nutrition or minerals in them.

Here is a food plan according to Dr. Bernard Jensen, a pioneer in nutrition who wrote several books on this topic.

In his best book, *Vibrant Health from Your Kitchen,* he points out that 80% of the nutrients in the blood are alkaline and 20% are acidic. To preserve the blood balance, we need to know which foods are alkaline and which are acidic. Most vegetables are alkaline, protein and starches (carbohydrates) are acidic. Six vegetables and two fruits make up that 80% of alkaline foods we need, while protein and starches (carbs) are 20% of acidic foods. This makes sense to me. This means more vegetables, less of the other foods. Genius!

This is the food section of the book. I am literally going to bombard you with foods you never dreamed of before we started.

Alkalinity in the body is very important to good health, and is a defense against disease and death.

The following lists[3], from Ragnar Berg of Germany, indicate foods creating alkalinity in the body and those generating acid in the body.

[3] Source - www.nacd.org

Column 1	Column 2	Column 3
Alkaline-Forming Non Starch Foods	**Alkaline-Forming Proteins and Fruits**	**Alkaline-Forming Starchy Foods**
alfalfa, artichokes, asparagus, string and wax beans, whole beets, beet leaves, broccoli, white and red cabbage, carrots, carrot tops, cauliflower, celery knobs, chicory, coconut, corn, cucumbers, dandelions, eggplant, endive, garlic, horse-radish, kale, kohlrabi, leek, lettuce, mushrooms, okra, ripe olives, onions, oster plant, parsley, parsnips, fresh peas, sweet peppers, radishes, rutabagas, savory, sea lettuce, sorrel, soy bean (products), spinach, sprouts, summer squash, swiss chard, turnip, watercress	apples, apricots, avocados, cantaloupes, cranberries, currents, dates, figs, grapes, grapefruit, lemons, limes, oranges, peaches, pears, persimmons, pineapple, plums, prunes, raisins, rhubarb, tomatoes	bananas, white potatoes, pumpkin, hubbard squash
	Acid-Forming Proteins and Fruits	**Acid-Forming Starchy Foods:**
	beef, buttermilk, chicken, clams, cottage cheese, crab, duck, eggs, goose, fish, honey (pure), jello, lamb, lobster, mutton, nuts, oysters, pork, rabbit, raw sugar, turkey, turtle, veal	barley, lima and white beans, bread, cereal, chestnuts, corn, cornmeal, cornstarch, crackers, grapefruit, gluten flour, lentils, macaroni, maize, millet rye, oatmeal, peanuts, peanut butter, dried peas, brown and polished rice, roman meal, rye flour, sauerkraut, tapioca

Combine foods from columns one and two, and also from one and three. **Avoid combinations from columns two and three.**

Learn to balance your blood. Our blood is 80% alkaline and 20% acid. We need to learn about portions, and remember the 6-2-1-1 formula:

6	vegetables	60%
2	fruits	20%
1	protein	10%
1	carbohydrate	10%
	Total	100%

Did you know?[4]....

- Too much sugar can break down your immune system; 1 teaspoon can crash the immune system for 6 hours?
- A woman in her lifetime will use four to five pounds of lipstick?
- A single peanut contains 183 different pesticides?
- Coffee has 200+ chemicals? (make sure it's organic)
- The second largest ingredient in salt is sugar?
- Seedless watermelons and grapes are GMO?
- A healthy liver takes twelve weeks to process a deep fried food?
- An English cucumber grows in twelve hours with chemicals?
- The majority of North American breweries use low quality ingredients and very minimum fermentation? In order to make it palatable, they convince you to drink it ice cold. In English pubs, they brew it fresh and warm.
- One cigarette contains several thousand chemicals?
- A female in Canada age 19 to 30 uses 100 pounds of sugar yearly?
- Males in Canada uses age 30 to 50 uses 85 pounds of sugar yearly?
- Every Monday, 40 million Americans and 2 million Canadians go on a diet?
- That on this planet, there are more than 1,800 volcanos?
- Organic food is escalating 30% per year? (This is good news!)
- The USA is #36 on obesity? (Americans, do something about it!)
- All corn and soya beans are GMO?
- Sugar beets are GMO?
- Some bananas are GMO?
- Papaya grown in Hawaii are GMO?
- The word ORGANICS has been claimed and copyrighted by Loblaw?# (Is it fair that the copyright office let this happen?)
- The word MILK has been claimed by the dairy industry and trademarked and you cannot use it at all for any reason?
- Your large intestine, the colon, holds a maximum of four meals at one time and the fifth meal must be evacuated?

---

[4] This information was collected from various magazines and stats.

- North American farmers currently use approximately 900 Million pounds of pesticides and 22 billion pounds of synthetic fertilizers, fungicides herbicides and growth regulator fumigants to protect foods while they are in transit?
- When you dig out worms from the ground to go fishing, you hurt the soil's natural process to fertilize the seeds?
- Our governments prefer a dumber society, so they are able to control us better?
- Retirees at 65 die at 67 for lack of dreams? (So. continue to dream, people, or find a dream.)
- According to scientists a bumble bee's body weight is too heavy to fly? (Someone forgot to tell the bumble bee.)
- A young couple freshly married will divorce after 3 years? (Who knows why, maybe for lack of dedication?)

Notes

Chapter 11

CLEANSING AND REBUILDING

Your body will cleanse for you each and every day, with or without your permission. Somehow, there is a blueprint in us that knows how to deal with our challenges. Did you ever cut your finger, for example? Yes, of course you did. It didn't heal by itself, but if you kept it dirty, it would get infected. You had to make an effort to keep the wound free of dirt and germs.

Your insides are the same. The organs get sluggish if we don't cleanse each and every day. We must consume water. How much water? In general, doctors say 6 large glasses or the equivalent of 1.5 litres of water is crucial. When you wash your dishes or laundry or floors, you must use water, not pop or coffee. When it rains, it doesn't rain coffee or pop. I am being silly about it, but it seems like so many people don't know what water is in our country. We don't have to be like camels, their excuse is that there is no water in the desert.

The best bath a person can have is a salt water one. Sodium is considered the youth element. Studies have shown people with a high intake of natural sodium have better bowels, a youthful look and vibrant health. I speak for myself.

**If you lost your sense of humor, start eating organic foods.
With the extra nutrients you might get your humor back.**
– Paul Ciaravella

For these people, it does not matter what climate they are in, southwest USA or eastern USA; in both climates, they perspire and they will have a loss of sodium. This mineral is very important. You can balance this by eating strawberries, celery, the whites of eggs, put a pinch of sea salt in your glass of water, also the white of the water melon (don't throw it out, it is gold for your body) and also potato peels. Eat these and you will be taking better care of yourself by bringing more alkalinity to your body.

The Dry Body - I am a dry body, skinny with no fat. This is the reason we call it dry. High in metabolism with a very good appetite and dry skin. Sometimes we feel cold, we are sports minded and active. I have analyzed the population. A large number of Orientals are dry bodies. Their diet consists of vegetables and garlic, a good balance which is easier to digest. If you can't have garlic, try one of the other foods like onions.

The Damp Body - This type of body is very common in our society. 65% of women are born with damp bodies, both black and white. Orientals are about 15%, because the past generation mainly ate vegetables. Obesity is going through the roof. This body type has to be careful.

The 5 symptoms can include obesity; sugar cravings; eating mainly carbohydrates, grains, sugars, beverages and sweets.

Should you have this condition, here is the answer to dry up the body. Since sugars and carbohydrates are wet foods, and if you eat them, you are going to get wetter (fat), you should stay away from these foods.

Here is a plan for each body type

Hot body - cool off the body; eat less hot foods listed above.

Cold body - eat more of the hot foods listed above.

Dry body - since you have good metabolic system, balance your foods; eat 50 /50 listed above.

Damp body - you are the challenge A damp body is considered wet if you eat wet foods (wet foods = more fat) to dry up your body

1) Eat 7 vegetables daily, you can juice as well.
2) To dry up your body, use fresh herbs daily and you will have a balance.
3) Eat 2 to 3 fruits daily, must be classified organic.
4) Eat only 1 carbohydrate daily.
5) Eat only 1 protein daily.
6) Drink between meals, put a pinch of sea salt in your water.
7) Buy and eat more organic and whole foods
8) Make sure to invite oils and fats into your body, such as olive, coconut, pumpkinseed, flax (but not canola it is a GMO oil).
9) Introduce exercise, the best is to walk every day.
10) Eat more yellow foods for better bowel movements.
11) Take better care of your colon than you do your car.

These are the 11 simple commandments to stay vibrant and healthy.

I make no claims; the body type method has been here in our society for many years. For a better and healthier life style, I understand them and I personally use them.

People feel hot and cold in the world. Canada is cold and hot and damp but not dry. Asia is damp and hot. Africa is hot and dry. Australia is cold and hot. The US Southwest is dry and the east is cold and hot and damp. Florida is damp and hot.

Find your climate. If you are challenged, you can move to the climate you prefer. (By the way, you can move around Trees cant.)

Every Monday morning, 40 million Americans go on a weight loss program. In Canada, with our lower population, 2 million Canadians start a diet

They don't have the information you have right now.

Chapter 12

CO-FACTORS

Organic foods have more minerals and vitamins than conventional foods. Co-factors are the dream of the entire body. Basically, it is the foundation of nutrition.

For example, if you eat a meal without the co-factors, then the body has to borrow from itself to process this meal. It is very important that we know this or otherwise we rob ourselves of nutrition, we will be starving and the cravings will go out of control. Not only will you crave but you'll be tired, cranky and negative all the time. I know, I have been there myself. There is a chart of co-factors in a previous chapter on organic farming.

Study this information. This book is not only for organics. It is also to understand how the body assimilates foods. Why do we chew our foods, and what is the enzyme ptyalin for and where does it come from? It comes from saliva. When you eat raw foods, you chew to moisten them and grind them. Besides that, your jaw will get stronger and also supply the digestive system with much-needed roughage that helps the bowel tone itself.

We need to strengthen our blood. Some foods are blood builders; the herb nettle is a wonderful blood builder, also, beets, green vegetables, black cherries, bee pollen and chlorella. All of these are excellent blood builders. Some foods are brain foods that nourish the brain with phosphorus-rich foods. The same foods that feed the brain will nourish the nerves and the glands. We also need fats for the brain because fats are what heat the body.

I am extremely passionate about this information having to deal with Parkinson's personally.

Food cravings and moods each organ has a different job to perform. The kidneys don't perform the same work that the liver does, ditto the lungs. According to the chemical structure that determines its function, the necessary chemicals are brought to them by the bloodstream. They say that our blood is the river of life.

Meats are very destructive to our wellbeing. We often turn to sweets, especially those men who bring candy to their wife or girlfriend. But sweetness is also found in raw honey in pies and cakes. This affection that we feel for our sweethearts can be a huge problem, but this problem can be corrected and the excess weight will come off via discipline. Pay attention to constipation, you have to get rid of it or your organs will be sluggish and therefore, your entire wellbeing will be sluggish.

Sugar flirts I find these relate to how much sugar we consume annually.

1) I have a sweet tooth
2) She has a sweet tooth
3) I have a sugar craving
4) They are sweet
5) My sweet heart
6) You are very sweet, thank you
7) She is so sweet
8) Hello honey
9) The second ingredient in salt is sugar
10) Honey, can you get me a cup of sugar
11) I take my coffee with 2 teaspoons of sugar
12) Sugar baby
13) Hello sweetie pie
14) you are my candy girl

How much sugar do you consume every year?

If you are age....

....9-13 – 115 pounds per year
....14-18 – 120 pounds per year
....19-30 – 100 pounds per year
....31 -50 – 85 pounds per year

Canadian stats call for 100 pounds each annually! We are breaking down our immune system going to the coffee shops with your car ... and, think of the fuel being used.

The American stats call for 1200 teaspoon annually per person, a little bit higher.

Did you know that a teaspoon of white sugar will break down your immune system for at least 6 hours? If each person uses roughly 100 pounds a year, that's a lot of immune system break down!

Chapter 13

NUTRITION

Nutrition Everybody talks about it. What does it mean? In my case, I get a pain in my gut that feels like I am hungry. Simple as that. What else can it be? At the same time, I get an urge to answer a natural call. What can it be, a bowel movement? Listen up...your body is talking to you. My foods are simple. I try organic as much as possible.

My nutrition I have three meals a day with two snacks between meals. I try to drink water as much as possible along with supplements. Always take your supplements early in the day, so they can be assimilated during the day.

Foods are key in this order:

Greens - Kale - celery - lettuce - beet tops - spinach, this combo has Sodium chlorine, excellent cleansers. Make a salad. Collards - fennel - cabbage - Brussels sprouts - avocado - asparagus - parsley - endive - escarole - green figs - chicory - celery root - broccoli - artichoke - dandelion - Swiss chard - okra - green beans, Greens build your bones.

Yellows - These foods are semi laxatives - beans - squash - millet - peppers - mangos - bananas - Yellow polenta - egg yolk - pineapple - peaches - apricots yellow beets.

Reds - These foods stimulate the organs - peppers - cabbage - beets - pomegranates - tomatoes - pumpkin - red onion - red grapes - cherries - strawberries - raspberries -red potatoes - radicchio - red figs.

These are some of the foods that we should eat; they are also available at most of the organic restaurants, health food stores and organic weekend markets.

Steps to healthy well being

Step 1 We have to chew each mouthful of food twenty times; this way we have plenty of saliva to process this organic meal.

Step 2 The food should organic. If you should have a mental health challenge, you will be safe from lethal chemicals that can cause trouble.

Step 3 Don't drink with your meals or otherwise you will invite indigestion. It is like getting a hose and washing out most of the digestive enzymes. Wait 35 minutes, then drink. Remember, in fast food restaurants, when they sell you a meal, combo #1 has a drink, so does #2, #3 and so on. The drinks are only sugar and ice and you won't be able to process that meal. The sugar will alter the gut acid and you will experience heart burn. Just try it.

Step 4 If it is organic, our food contains co-factors. What are they? They are minerals and vitamins our body stores; from Vitamin A to Z, calcium, to iron, to sodium, all of When the body is in need, secretions go to the colon and to the liver. Here is the catch and why we have to learn nutrition. Should you eat a non-organic dinner, it will be very low in co-factors, then the body has to secrete cofactors from its own body to secure digestion. You don't want to destroy that beautiful meal. Basically, you have robbed Peter to pay Paul; this is the most important lesson to a better education on being vibrant and nutritionally healthy.

Supplements Why should I take them? I am eating organic, shouldn't that be enough? Well, yes and no. Some soils don't have all the minerals. To be sure, take a multivitamin, some digestive enzymes, and avoid indigestion at all costs.

The other smart thing to do is to rotate your foods. For example, the next time you shop, buy potatoes from Utah, the time after, from Prince Edward Island, following that, Idaho. You see what I am saying? By rotating different origins, you get a bit of minerals from each soil from that location. The same goes for apples, oranges, bananas, all foods. You will become a smarter consumer. But sometimes, we get lazy, we are in our comfort zone and we forget. If your doctor knew these things, he or she would remind you, but is not his or her job; it is yours.

I am organic in my heart, but sometimes it is not possible to be one. Off season, stores don't have as much in their inventory as farmers are unable to grow as much. In season, yes, I can say very loudly, I am eating my way to vibrant health. We have multiple countries to choose from. Ask your local organic store to let you know the rotation of foods. One week from Europe; one week from South America; in seasons, buy from Ontario and California and so on. It is very helpful to gather nutrition from various other countries.

Just because it is organic doesn't mean it's good for you. For instance, if you are diabetic and you eat many organic carbohydrates, you are going to need a lot of insulin to break them down. Be wise; respect the research that has been done in the past by professionals. All right; find the foods that fit your life style. And health requirement.

Some people say, I don't know what to eat. Here is a small list of some of the foods to choose from. I list them for you to choose.

Berries	Greens	Fruits
Blackberry, blueberry, cheriy, cranberry, elderberry, hucklebeny, mulberry, raspberry, strawbeny, gooseberry	Artichoke, asparagus, broccoli, Brussels sprouts, cabbage, celery root, chicory, collards, dandelion, endive, escarole, kale, lettuce, parsley, spinach, Swiss chard, watercress	Apple, apricot, avocado, banana, dates, figs, grapes, grapefruit, guava, mango, melons, nectarine, orange, papaya, peach, pear, persimmon, tangerine, pineapple, plum

Have you noticed in the last ten years, there so many more seedless fruits oranges watermelon grapes? Seeds are key to help nourish the glands and help the brain, and nervous system. People are having sex imbalances, problems in the brain and reproductive issues which can be mitigated with the proper nutrients found in seeds. Our next generation depends on these seeds. It is sad, these seeds have all the chemical elements and nucleic acids to produce new life.

Berries Almost all berries have a laxative effect. Most people eat the red part of the watermelon, but the white part has sodium, which is good for your joints. You can also eat the seeds (if you can find watermelon with seeds... good luck, this has become a seedless world.)

Strawberries are among the highest fruits in sodium. (Even the "Beatles" agree that strawberry fields are forever.) Mulberries have an unusual taste, but they are very good for the stomach walls and help with ulcers. Persimmon, I have been eating most of my life, I consider them lifelong fruits.

Pumpkin seeds, they are good for the prostate and also high in alkaline.

The foods mentioned are for health and well-being.

All salted foods, giant food processors of crackers, nuts, popcorn, and salted seeds are bad foods. This group of foods are constipating, including coffee, cheese, some vinegars, chocolate and burned foods. I say stay away from them.

"The 3 Worst Foods"

Rhubarb It is high in oxalic acid and adds to your aching joints.
Cranberries You have to eat them cooked - very high in oxalic acid.
Green plums This is another food that will cause stomach aches - avoid.

According to the lore of these three foods, Native Americans watched what birds ate; they didn't even get close to the tree if the birds didn't want to. Why should we? Just something to think about.

Great foods

Eggs have great nutrients for the brain. Since my diagnosis with Parkinson's, I jumped on that fact. They help my nerves glands and brain and also have lecithin which helps with production in the sex organs. I take all I can get.

Sodium, the youth element there are a number of sources of sodium:

1) Sodium chloride - it is manmade, and the second largest ingredient is sugar
2) Animals - the white of the egg is very high in sodium
3) Sea salts - come from Earth Mountains
4) Black lava salt (my favorite) from Iceland - high in energy
5) Fruits and vegetables

We need all we can get. Be wise, stay away from sodium chloride. Consume all of the others, Sodium builds strength. The more sodium the tissue takes up, the more alkaline and stronger they become. A deficiency of sodium starves the inner organs. Too much calcium can get in the way of the joints, then we invites other problems.

A strong person has the proper foods.

Good sources of sodium - egg whites, chicken, turkey, red cabbage, apples, barley, watermelon bottoms, asparagus, collard greens, dandelions, figs, strawberries, seaweed, horseradish, Irish moss, raw cow's milk, kale, celery, kelp, mustard greens, black olives, okra, veal joint broth, potato peels, Swiss chard, whey, sunflower seeds, sesame seeds, spinach, celery root, raisins, water chestnuts, radishes, broccoli, Brussels sprouts, cashews and miso.

Calcium sodium A personal story to share.... my mother had a car accident as a passenger. She broke her upper arm in three places. You have to give her credit, at the time, she was 84 years old. I encouraged her to eat more greens and she had speedier results. When we went to see the doctor three weeks after the accident, the doctor could not believe it. On the x-ray, her arm looked almost healed. We were shocked that a person of her age could heal so quickly. Greens make a difference, big time. The doctor was so impressed that he asked me for permission to display her x- ray in the national archive. I said yes, of course. On the way home, my mother asked me what the doctor was talking about and I replied that she was his best patient ever.

Use gelatine to increase your calcium. Gelatin is fabulous to increase calcium intake as gelatin is actually 48% calcium. To prepare it, use cherry or strawberry juice to give it a little sweet taste and avoid sugar. Medicine can be in your food (food is your medicine, medicines are food).

Some opinions about foods...

I rank biodynamic foods top of the list along with organic foods as long they are local and fresh and away from pesticides. Should they travel from thousands of miles away, they are not fresh.

Oxtails

One of key foods who knows how long this food has been around,
Jamaicans love this dish
I learned to make this dish over the years the reason why I call it key
food it has healing property 'is the one
The meat is good too lets make it.

4 to 6 small pieces of ox tails
A fair size pot 2 litres of water
Bring to a boil for approx. 1 hour slow heat
1 red onion I fennel 1 celery root
Add to the ox tails for another hour
Now add table spoon turmeric tea spoon sea salt
Tea spoon cayenne pepper table spoon of sage
Tea spoon of oregano
Greens 2 leafs kale 2 collards and spinach
Combined cooking 2/1/2 hours if low in water
Add some this broth helps with the lymph the
Sex organs and overall the wellbeing it is
One of my favourite do not change the formula
Some chefs add red pepper tomato sauce remember
The broth has healing properties no claims made.
Paul Ciaravella

Notes

Ingredients

4 to 6 pieces of ox tales
2 litres of water
1 red 1 white onion
1 fennel
1 celery root
1 table spoon turmeric
1 table spoon of sea salt
1 tea spoon of cayenne pepper
1 tablespoon sage
Use any type of greens
Greens collards any kale leafs
What ever greens you have

Paul Ciaravella

Breakfast - 7:30 am
Fruits, cereal, almond milk
Coconut oil spread on toast
1 egg, poached scrambled
Hand full of almonds, (make sure they were soaked
Overnight and chew them well)
Tea (use 7x7 Alkaherb from Dr. P. Jentshura)

Lunch - 12 pm
Squash soup or carrot or potatoes
Cut up 2 stems of kale and put them in the soup
Do not throw out potatoes peels use them in your soup
Pumpkinseed oil, sea salt, bok choy
Sandwich of your choice
Finish with celery sticks and raw bok choy.

Dinner - 6 pm
Roast lamb or turkey
Serve with asparagus, carrots and green vegetables
Brown rice or wild rice (pour some Coconut oil on the rice,
for spice use turmeric)
**A good hearty meal was introduced to you by someone
for you to enjoy; return the favour.
Eat guilt free.**

This chili recipe was created by Paul Ciaravella in 2013. It is very tasty and nutritious. It has all the fats, proteins, vegetables, herbs, spices and sulfur needed by your body. It helps with the heat and the sea salts give you minerals. Should you be battling Parkinson's, this food is for you.

Black bean chili with coconut oil and coconut milk

1/4 cup (60 ml) coconut oil
2 lb. (900 g) lean ground beef*
2 red onions, chopped
1 red bell pepper, chopped
3/4 cup (185 mL) chopped, mixed fresh herbs (rosemary, oregano, sage)
1 tsp. (5 mL) each, fine sea salt, cayenne pepper
Pinch of ground ginger
Two, 28-oz (796-mL) cans crushed or diced tomatoes
Two, 19-oz (540-mL) cans black beans, rinsed, drained 398-mL cans coconut milk
Heat oil in a large sauce pan over medium high until melted. Add beef, cook stirring for 10 minutes. Add onions, red peppers and herbs. Cook stirring for 5 minutes and stir in salt, cayenne and ginger. Add tomatoes, beans and coconut milk. Stir well. Bring to a boil and reduce heat to medium-low. Cover and simmer 1 to 2 hours to let the flavors develop. Makes about 12 cups (3 1), if too much, use half the recipe.
*You can make it vegetarian, just leave out the beef, if 11 come out just as good.
Sicilian Frittata (This can be a meal anytime of the day)
Small fraying pan 12 inches with lid
5 eggs
4 oz. fresh ricotta
1 small zucchini, chopped the size of a dime
4 small red potatoes, chopped
1 red pepper, chopped
6 stems asparagus, chopped
1 red onion, chopped
2 tablespoons coconut oil
When the ground is dry nothing will grow; no plants will survive, so drink some water before you dry up too. Our country has plenty of water.
Between meals, drink water and make sure it is filtered.

Once you had master chef for a tutor; the food was cooked to death. Then you met a nutritionist, who said to put a seed into a hot oven for 2 minutes, then pull it out and sow it in soil. Would it grow? Of course not? The seed is dead; the enzymes are no longer active. No deal.
- Paul Ciaravella

ACKNOWLEDGMENTS

I would like to thank the following professionals for their input:

Dr. Bernard Jensen, Nutritionist, Author, Chiropractor,
David Roland, PhD, Nutritionist Corola Barzak, Nutritionist
Dr. Doris J. Rapp, MD, FAAA, FAAP, environmental medical specialist
and pediatric allergist
Deborah A Drake, B.Sc., .MD (retired), N.H.P., CBS, food and chemistry
expert
Elaine Gottschalk, Author, biochemist and cell biologist Eric Marsden,
BSC, ND
Dr. Koontz, MD
Hamad Aboukhazaal, Master Herbalist, source of knowledge, experience
and wisdom
Dr Zoltán P. Rona, ND, Author
Richard Chomko, media photographer
Mary Cento, photographer, Cento studio, photographer
Michael Schmidt, Biodynamic farmer
Mike Lanigan, Biodynamic farmer
Joe Bom, Biodynamic farmer (deceased)
Tomas Nimmo, Guelph Organic Conference
Teresa Ciaravella, School Trustee, Maple Schools
Lorna Eaton, Editor

RECOMMENDED READING

Vibrant Health from Your Kitchen, Dr. Bernard Jensen

Tissue Cleansing Thru Bowel Management, 1981, Dr. Bernard Jensen

Foods that Heal, 1988, Dr. Bernard Jensen

Nature has a Remedy, 1979, Dr. Bernard Jensen

Come Alive, 1979, Dr. Bernard Jensen

Food Healing for Man, 1983, Dr. Bernard Jensen

The Wheel of Health: The Sources of Long Life and Health Among the Hunza, 2006, Dr. G. T. Wrench, MD

Chlorella the Jewel of the Far East, 1992, Dr. Bernard Jensen

Guess What came to Dinner: Parasites and Your Health, Ann Louise Gittleman, PhD, CNS, 2001

Doctor Patient Handbook, 1978, Dr. Bernard Jensen

The Joy of Living and How to Attain it, 1946, Dr. Bernard Jensen

Pottenger's Cats - A Study in Nutrition, 1983, Francis M. Pottenger, Jr., MD

Nutrition and Physical Degeneration, 2008, Weston A. Price

The Cure is in the Cupboard, 2009, Dr. Cass Ingram

The Healing Foods, 1992, Patricia Hausmaun and Judith Benn Hurley

The Raw Food Detox Diet, 2006, Natalia Rose

Candida Silver Mercury Fillings and the Immune System, Helyn Luechauer DDS

Healing without Medication, 2015, Robert S. Rister

The Illustrated Encyclopedia of Healing Remedies, 1998, C. Norman Shealy

The Cure for all Diseases, 1995, Hulda Clark, PhD ND

Is this your Child's World: A Wakeup Call, 1996, Doris J. Rapp, MD

Holistic Nutrition, Canadian Nutrition Institute Inc.

Beauty to Die For, 1991 Judi Vance

The Nutrition Desk Reference, 1998, Robert Garrison, MD, Elizabeth Somer, M.A.

Breaking the Vicious Cycle, 1994, Elaine Gottschalk

Holistic Herbal, 2013, David Hoffmann

Discovering the Human Body, 1992, Bernard Knight. MD
Diet for a New America, 1987, Dr. John Robbins
Chemistry made Simple, 1984, Fred C. Hess, ED.D
At Home with Herbs, 1994, Jane Newdick
Nutritional Influences on Illness, 1997, Melvyn R. Werbach, MD
Ending Denial, 2013, Helke Ferrie
The Magic of Thinking Big, 1987, David J Schwartz
See You at the Top, 2009, Zig Ziglar
Think and Grow Rich, 1937, Napoleon Hill
The Law of Success, 1925, Napoleon Hill

**Farmers get up early with the roosters
singing. They work long hours for us.
Give them a chance. One time someone
gave you a chance - buy local.
May the power of nutrition be with you always and stay vibrant**
-Paul Ciaravella

People and plants, trees, grass, animals, fruits, vegetables and fish, water and so on require nutrients and oxygen. It is shocking that we have lost more than 40% of our oxygen in the atmosphere also we have depleted our soils.

The kale picture listed here was grown with Paramagnetic rock in my back yard. These plants grew more than 6 feet tall. The rest of the vegetables, looked so vibrant and healthy, and they were tasty. The magnetic rock was an idea that me and some friends thought of. We got a volcanic rock and ground it into sand form and spread it in our garden. Our plants grew better. The evidence is here. Try some of the Paramagnetic rock.

PAUL was born in the southern part of Italy where the weather is warm and the fruits taste great, in 1987 Paul took an interest in learning all he could about nutrition with great desire to be a nutritionist and to have a vibrant body.